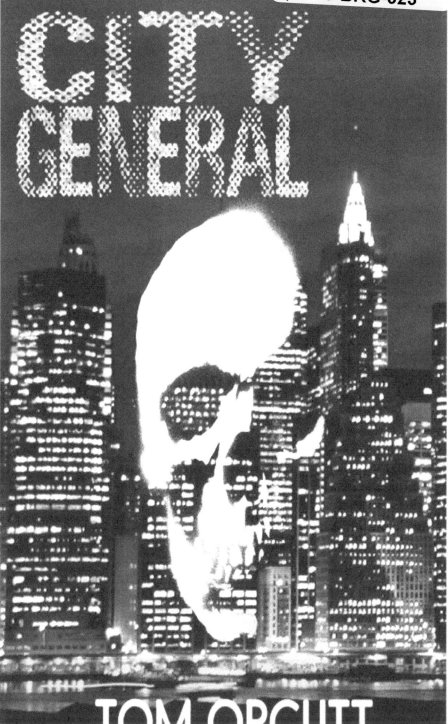

CITY GENERAL

TOM ORCUTT

City General

Written By Tom Orcutt

S haron

enjoy!

Tom Orcutt

ISBN: 978-1-7350485-0-5

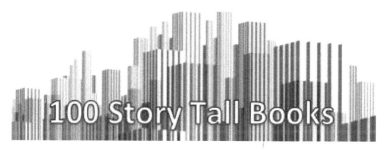

100 Story Tall Books

Dedication

This book is dedicated to my late wife Holly, whose inspiration and motivation to compile these stories and complete this project was awesome. I miss you!

City General

Disclaimer

Introduction

Rape, murder, sex, drugs, gambling, theft, shootings, stabbings...

These are incidents you don't want to hear about before entering a hospital, either as a visitor, or patient.

Could you survive City General?

Turn the pages and wander
the halls if you dare...

Sexual Harassment

"If only all of the workplace sexual harassment laws put into place in the 1990s had existed in the 1980s...I would probably be rich", Molly H. thought to herself, after quite an eventful day in the operating room.

An operating room is a bustling and hustling place. From the scrub room outside, to the actual procedure, and then the clean-up afterwards, these rooms are quite busy on a daily basis. Patients go in, patients live, patients die, babies are born, babies are murdered, quite a variety of events unfold, either planned or unplanned.

Molly H. was finishing up her nursing school education. As part of her clinical education, she had to go through various "rotations"... a few weeks working with psych patients, orthopedics, a general "med-surg" floor, and then an actual surgical rotation-assisting and helping the surgeon in whatever capacity was needed. Though she had witnessed autopsies and watched videos of surgical procedures, this was to be her first real case in an actual operating room.

Mr. Gavin was the patient. A sixty-seven-year-old man, who had developed prostate cancer. Many medical experts feel that all men will develop this disease if they "live long enough". The procedure today was to "open the patient up"-by opening his lower abdomen, exposing the prostate, and then to implant some radioactive "seeds" which would destroy the cancer cells that were present.

The surgeon today was Dr. Mendenhall, a urologist who had been practicing for many years and was well known in this Catholic institution of healing. He was always boisterous, and usually obnoxious. However, he had been there so long, that he thought he could pretty much say and do as he pleased.

Molly was married, happy, and just wanted to finish up her studies and graduate. She had just slipped out of her student uniform and put on scrubs. Her pretty red hair was tucked into her surgical cap and her smile was hidden by the surgical mask. As she entered the operating room, she saw that the patient was already sedated and asleep. She donned the surgical gloves and was ready to go...

"And who do I have the pleasure of working with today?" Dr. Mendenhall inquired.

"Molly H, ", she replied.

"Well, I want you to be working as close to me as possible-you'll be holding the retractors and keeping his belly opened".

"Sounds good," she responded.

As Molly moved closer to the patient, she double-checked, "Where exactly do you want me?"

"Why in bed, of course," the surgeon responded.

As the procedure continued, at one point he said, "It's very tempting to reach around you and fondle you, young lady."

She was embarrassed, but she also couldn't believe he would talk to her like that with so many nurses and staff around.

A few minutes passed.

"So, Molly, are you married?"

"Yes".

"Well I am too. I've been married for thirty years and I've had sex with my wife 3,658 times. But I can tell you one thing, if I were married to you, the number would be at least twice that, Hell, I bet we'd be pushing 10,000 times!"

Luckily, the surgical mask was hiding her embarrassment. She was speechless.

As the years passed by and the workplace harassment laws went into effect-Molly thought to herself and told her husband, "Where were these laws when we needed them? There were plenty of witnesses. We'd be rich!"

As a prologue/follow-up to this story, Molly and Dr. M. would cross paths again. Molly had the occasion of attending a wake of a well-known and well-liked radiology technician that had suddenly died. There were many hospital employees and physicians coming by to pay their respects.

As Molly was talking to another nurse, she noticed good ole Dr. Mendenhall enter the room. He glanced at her but there was no sign of recognition. Molly felt relieved and she remembered that during her last encounter, she was pretty much covered from head to toe.

The widow of the deceased was up front as expected, greeting and receiving condolences from the visitors. She was holding a baby, her first grandchild. Mendenhall approached.

"So, who do we have here?", he inquired.

"This is baby Kathleen," the widow replied.

"Well, she's a cutie. Better get her started on birth control pills now, because she's gonna have all the action she can handle!"

Molly, the widow, and others nearby couldn't believe what they had just heard...a crude, sexual remark about a newborn baby!

They all would have liked to clobber him. Dr. Mendenhall is still practicing today.

The Disappearance of Suzy Wilson

Suzy was an attractive 27-year-old who was having some emotional problems. There had been a lot of stress in her life lately. She had lost one parent to illness, endured a broken engagement, and was worried that someone was out to get her, that she "would be next".

Her regular physician referred her to a psychiatrist, who noted that alcohol and drugs were becoming a part of her daily routine. He suggested that she may benefit by some group and individual therapy, and that a short stay in a psychiatric ward may be beneficial to her.

She knew and conceded that "things weren't right", and she wanted to get better. After she checked with her employer and her insurance, she verified that she could indeed take some time off, and she saw this as a possible solution to her problems.

Unit 10 Assistance was the name of the floor and unit to which she would be admitted. "Psych ward" was no longer used as it was cold, and conjured up images of an old black-and-white movie, *The Snake Pit*, with Olivia de Havilland.

Hospital administration felt that an "Assistance Unit" sounded more friendly and this name would help incoming patients begin to immediately feel better.

Since the staff feared that Suzy may harm herself, she was put on the "locked side of the unit" - her patient room was not locked, but the doors to the unit were. Special keys were needed for hospital departments such as Food Service and Housekeeping to enter, and it was a very secure area. Patients were not allowed to leave the unit without being accompanied by staff.

Though Suzy had high expectations and wanted to get better, her paranoia increased and she wanted to escape. This became the focus of her existence.

Then, it happened. Suzy disappeared.

The staff discovered her missing shortly before noon. They scrambled looking at her chart, desperately hoping that she went with the staff to deliver something or go off the floor for a diagnostic medical test.

Other patient rooms were being checked-perhaps she was just visiting someone. No tests had been ordered; all patients were accounted for. Where was Suzy?

The chief of the Psychiatry department called the police. A few officers arrived on the scene and began to search, not only the "Unit 10 Assistance" floor, but the entire hospital.

Robert S. worked on the first floor of the hospital, in a rather small office, adjacent to an employee locker room. When he saw the police glancing into his office (which took all of two seconds), and then entering the locker room, he quipped, "What are you guys looking for, a body?"

"Yes! What do you know about this?", the policeman inquired.

Robert S. was taken aback by the question-after all, he thought he was just trying to be funny.

"I don't know anything!", he responded, now trying not to be regarded a suspect in Suzy's disappearance.

Police and hospital staff were scrambling everywhere-inside and outside. Charts were being checked, washrooms were being double-checked, but the time and hours of her disappearance were mounting. The anxiety and stress level of the employees, police, and administrators was going through the roof.

Then, out of nowhere, a maintenance man saw a possibility-a remote one at that, but yes, it was possible. A stark, cold steel door, about 24x24 provided the deadly answer to this puzzle.

On the 10th floor, not too far from the nursing station, was a door with a pull-down handle. The housekeeping staff used this door all the time, but to the rest of the employees on the floor, they were oblivious.

You see, what lay behind that door was a dark 10 story drop of a laundry chute into the basement. Unfortunately for Suzy, her neck broke and killed her during the fall, and her lifeless body was stuck between the second and third floor. The fire department was called to retrieve her body.

What happened after this tragedy? Locks were installed on all laundry chute doors, and only staff now held the keys.

"HELP!"

Being the Director of the Employee Relations/Human Resources Department of a large metropolitan hospital can be hazardous to your health.

Robert Stevens can attest to that. He had spent a long day dealing with hospital union negotiations, workman compensation cases, and meetings on how to hire and retain employees. The hospital was experiencing an employee turn-over rate of 3% per month. That doesn't sound bad, but that ultimately amounts to a 36% turn-over rate annually, which is unacceptable.

In the middle of this particularly hectic day, he had to squeeze in a few job interviews. He did interviews from time to time, but not on a daily basis. One of his staff was absent and he was thrust into doing a couple of preliminary screenings. Robert asked the interviewee how his attendance was at his previous position. With this question, the person dropped to the floor and proceeded to do 50 pushups just to prove, "I'm a healthy guy and never get sick".

This certainly caught Robert by surprise, but this wasn't to be the biggest surprise he would have today. He proceeded to call his wife and he told her that he was leaving soon, and about what had just happened in his office. They laughed, and then hung up. He threw some papers into an attaché case, turned the lights off, and proceeded to the parking garage.

In many major city hospitals, there are multi-level story parking garages for both visitors and staff. Robert got into an elevator, alone, and pushed the button for the 7th floor. He exited the elevator and saw his car sitting about 100 feet away.

As he was walking, he suddenly got shoved from behind and heard a voice, "Gimme your wallet!" Robert quickly turned around. He was confronted by a teen, approximately fifteen years old, brandishing a knife.

"Give me your wallet", he repeated, a little more forcefully.

Robert quickly assessed the situation. He stood about 6 feet 3 inches and weighed about 230. His attacker was a skinny kid, about 5 feet 7.

The knife was the "equalizer".

Fortunately, the knife wasn't a large hunting knife, but a folding pocket knife with a 4-inch blade. Not necessarily a life-threatening size, but it could certainly do some damage or kill you if it got placed in the wrong part of your body.

The kid made a threatening lunge at Robert.

"Give me your freakin' wallet!"

Robert blocked the assailants lunge with his attaché case.

"I'm not giving you anything!"

He did a quick assessment of his surroundings, and no one else was around. As he surveyed/assessed his situation, something caught the corner of his eye. A blue light. An escape! His assailant was getting more agitated and frustrated.

Placed in strategic places throughout the parking garage, there were emergency call stations indicated by a blue light. The idea was that if you were having car trouble, were lost, or "being the victim of a crime", you could press an emergency button and the hospital would immediately dispatch a security officer. This punky little kid stood between him and the light.

Robert started moving toward the knife-wielder, swung his attaché case once more, and then ran like Hell past him toward the emergency call button. The kid caught him, and another swipe was taken, but once more, it bounced off the attaché case. The assailant followed, but then he saw the light too. Just as he reached the emergency call box, Robert saw it...a small index card taped to the box. "Out of Order".

The assailant saw R.S. push the emergency button but failed to see the sign. He quickly assessed *his* situation, gave up, and bolted down the stairs and out of the garage.

The next morning there was an immediate meeting with the hospital President and Director of Security!

A Little Hanky Panky

Many doctors at teaching hospitals have two offices. There is one that is used to see and treat patients. If you are a department chairperson, you usually have another office in an "educational wing" of a building.

Dr. Rosen was an older, female Ob-Gyn doctor who had a nice office on the top floor of one particular building.

There were two parts to her office, an inner room with a desk and bookshelves, and an outer reception area. The outer room had a large window with blinds, and furnished with two chairs and a nice, "comfy-couch".

This office was in an area of the building with no patients, and fairly secluded. Her receptionist in this office, Diane, was a younger, attractive woman, who most males would not mind looking at.

My reason for going to, and being on that floor, was simple. There was a small auditorium on this floor, and part of my job was to set up and arrange equipment properly for upcoming meetings.

Well, let me just say that on several occasions, the blinds to Dr. Rosen's office were closed, and she and Diane were enjoying each other's company in extremely close proximately to one another!

I probably could have recorded what I heard, had I chosen to do so.

Oh well...let's just say that they were both consenting adults over 21. To each their own...

Something Smells Fishy

Security officer Zabroski worked as a patrolman for the hospital's security department. As a patrolman, he would respond to calls from the dispatcher via 2-way radios. In addition, he would routinely patrol certain areas of the hospital. The head of security would make out a weekly schedule, and to prevent boredom for the hospital patrolmen, they would rotate and cover different areas of the hospital complex.

Part of their responsibility were the parking lots-of which there were many. There were some outdoor, surface lots, and also a multi-story parking facility.

For the most part, Officer Zabrowski had to patrol these lots and make sure there was no loitering taking place, assist patrons who couldn't find their cars, help visitors who needed directions, etc.

Since this one parking lot was not an employee parking lot, cars were pretty much coming and going 24/7. If you did this job long enough, you would see the same car parked in different parts of the garage; repeat visitors. The job was pretty much routine and mundane, but absolutely necessary.

One car began to catch his eye-it was in the same place and hadn't been moved. Due to inactivity, after a few days it began showing signs of being dusty and dirty. Officer Zabrowski made a note of this, but after all, there were many simple explanations. It could belong to a hospitalized patient, or maybe broken down.

After about 5 days, with no notification from anyone regarding a disabled car, he contacted the local police department to "run the plates".

To his surprise, the car had been reported stolen from about 25 miles away. Officer Zabrowski took the hospital patrol car over to take a closer look. As he walked towards the car, he began to encounter a foul odor. With every step, the smell got worse and worse. He suddenly had a bad feeling about this. The smell was terrible.

Everything in the front seat looked in order. The back seat had a rug rolled up in it, and his flashlight saw some movement - small objects crawling on top of the rolled-up carpet.

At this point, he radioed his boss and got the ok to break into the car. After he broke a window and opened the vehicle's back door, the stench was overwhelming. He put a mask and gloves on and proceeded to pull the rug out. It was heavy, but he lowered it and set it on the ground, adjacent to the vehicle.

All of a sudden, he saw hair sticking out.

He called for help, and a medical crew was dispatched from the ER. A city policeman who happened to be in the ER on other business, accompanied the medical crew.

Those creepy-crawly objects that Officer Zabrowski saw on the rug?

Maggots!

As the rug was unrolled, the lifeless, decomposing body of a young woman was discovered. She was fully clothed, hands tied behind her back, and shot once in the head. The police and medical team opened the trunk, but it was empty. Someone had stolen this car 25 miles away, abducted this woman, killed her, and dumped the car and body and left them in this hospital parking lot.

The young woman was a missing college student from another part of the state. There should have been the opportunity for a lot of clues-but to this day the murder has not been solved. In addition, after a thorough check, there was absolutely no connection between the owner of the stolen car and the female victim.

The car was reported simply stolen from the owners' driveway, he had the keys, and there were no other keys found in the ignition or anywhere else in the car.

Frozen Peas

You would think that strangers wouldn't share intimate details of their lives with you the first time you meet.

It was my very first day at work at a prestigious medical center - my name badge proudly proclaimed the title, "Producer-Director".

I was getting the standard orientation for the building by my immediate supervisor, who took me around and introduced me to several people.

During this time, he made it clear to me that there are two, fifteen-minute breaks. He pointed out there was a usual group of people who met in the cafeteria during this time.

On my first break, there were about six of us, and my boss introduced me to the others around the table. Though this was my first "break" on my first day, they were a fun-loving, nice group of people, and I continued to meet with them daily for a long time.

One woman, an executive secretary to the head of nursing, Judie, decided to tell us about her husband.

"My hubby is off work today and in a lot of pain.", she said.

She proceeded to share that her husband had a vasectomy, the day before, and the doctor had to "fish around and look for the tubes to cut."

Yikes!

Unfortunately, (for him), she said, "His testicles are swollen and the size of a 16-inch-softball. He is sitting at home with two bags of peas on him, trying to get the swelling to go down."

Ouch!

It's Tinkle Tech Time!

Though the title of this segment is light-hearted, this is a serious situation that occurs at almost every hospital - just talk to the head of security at any hospital.

This happened to my boss. He was in the hospital as a patient, while I was working overtime editing a video project on a Saturday morning.

J.R. had fallen on the ice, and during the fall, his elbow had been shattered. He was hospitalized for almost a week. There was constant concern that small bone fragments might make their way into his bloodstream, so he was closely monitored and scanned.

Discharge time had finally arrived on a Saturday morning - he would be going home shortly. I was on an adjacent floor, listening to the mellow sounds of *Led Zeppelin* while editing a video. I was multi-tasking and way ahead of my time!

J.R. was lying in his bed, thinking about, and looking forward to his departure. His wife and kids would make the trip in to come pick him up.

Just then, a young man with a short, white lab coat walked into his room. He was wearing a stethoscope around his neck and holding a urine specimen cup.

"Hi! We need one more urine sample from you".

The young man in the lab coat handed J.R. the cup and motioned towards the bathroom. J.R. got up, took the cup, went into the washroom and closed the door. When he exited the bathroom holding the cup, he saw that his whole world had been invaded and changed!

The drawers to the night stand were all sitting open, his attaché case was gone, as well as his watch. J.R. ran out into the hallway, but the perpetrator was already gone…all in about three minutes.

After filing a security report, giving a description, and being discharged, he came down to where I was working (our offices were in the same area), and told me this exact story.

As a result, I was requested to create a video to be seen by all patients in the hospital.

The "Tinkle Tech" was not wearing a hospital issued I.D. badge…but he was wearing hospital-appropriate attire.

Patients were advised to check everyone who entered their room and look for proper identification. Darn impostors!

I Killed 19 People!

As video technology progressed over the years, my hospital department was given a generous donation to purchase color video cameras and new recording equipment. Up till then...I had black and white studio-type cameras which were very cool at the time, but this was an opportunity to upgrade to color.

Down the street from the hospital, there was a "broadcasting school" that offered a variety of television production and editing classes.

The school was in the market for some studio cameras for their basic fundamental classes. I ended up selling the old equipment to them, and as part of the negotiations over price, I was able to talk them into letting me take an advanced class I was interested in...for free.

After working full-time, this class met 4 nights a week, from 6 p.m. to 10 p.m. I talked myself into the fact that this would only be for 40 days, or 10 weeks, and that I could do this!

At this point in time, I was using a rapid transit system to commute to and from work. It was similar to the Metra in Washington, D.C., or what they call the CTA or "L" trains in Chicago.

During non-rush hours, the trains were relatively short, but they still ran every couple of minutes.

After night-school let out, I had a short, safe walk to catch a train. Now, late at night, and especially after 10 p.m., not all of the train cars were operational. They may have only two cars with the lights on…maybe less.

This particular night, only the front car of the train had the lights on and was in-service. There was the engineer/driver enclosed "box" in the right front corner, and as I entered the car, I noticed that there were only about 12 passengers on this train. Pretty much the usual amount for this time of night.

After a long day and night, I was relaxing and looking out the window, while others were reading or trying to sleep. We had made a few momentary scheduled stops, with people getting on, and people getting off.

Then…it happened.

A middle-aged man stood up and began his monologue. "You know…the police are so stupid. Over the last several years, I have killed 19 people. I shot some, stabbed some, and even strangled a few."

He was walking back and forth, up and down the aisle of the train.

As you can imagine, he got my attention, and my fellow riders' attention, right away.

"The police are stupid. They have never figured it out and come after me. I'm not in a very good mood tonight."

As I looked around at the other passengers, I was astonished that some people pretended to be asleep, others ignored him and continued to read.

I guess we all have our own reactions to stress!

Mine was different. My adrenal glands had kicked in and my body had entered the fight or flight reflex. The problem was there was no escape for the "flight reflex" part. I couldn't believe the passengers reactions.

I decided very quickly that I wasn't going to become his 20th victim! I wasn't going to just sit there and let him walk up and down the aisle and start hurting people. When and if he started to "make his move", I decided to lunge at him and try to protect myself and the others!

If I was going to die that night, I was going to go down swinging, and not just sit there and passively die! Believe me, I am no macho-man, my courage was coming from those pesky adrenal glands. I did know enough not to make direct eye contact...especially with a madman.

"The police are so stupid!", he re-iterated.

He had just walked past me, with his back to me, and then he made his move.

He put his hand in his pocket and pulled something out. He was still facing the other way.

All I could see was whatever he was holding had a long, black edge. From my viewpoint, it looked like the barrel of a handgun. I thought to myself, looks like this is it! Time to take this guy down.

It was all over in about 3 seconds.

The passengers and I had paid no attention to our moving train and we had no idea where we were. The stranger's actions had kind of gotten all our attention. Just as he started to turn around, the train pulled into a stop. In a flash, two policemen stepped in the door. They each grabbed one of his arms and he was off the train in a second.

As a prologue to this incident, it is interesting to hear how this potential deadly incident was averted. The quick-thinking engineer told us his story.

The engineer, using a mirror, saw the man walking up and down the aisle. The speakers in the train that announce the upcoming stops and stations, with the flip of a switch, turn into microphones. The engineer heard him talking about killing 19 people, and immediately radioed the police.

The police met the train at the next stop and when the doors opened, the perpetrator and passengers were totally surprised.

Luckily, no one was hurt.

We will never quite know what this man's story was...but it took quite a while for my adrenal glands to return to their normalcy, and for me to fall asleep that night!

If Only She Knew

Whether or not you feel abortion should remain legal is your personal decision.

However, abortion is the "legal" murder of an unborn baby - in a variety of gruesome ways, I might add.

One of the hospitals I worked at was going to remodel and update their OB floor. They decided to set up some focus groups to get some ideas and suggestions. Several women were contacted who had babies at the hospital over the past three years.

My job was to videotape these focus groups, so that the women's responses could be reviewed by staff, and their suggestions could be implemented.

One particular woman had nothing bad to say. After all, Dr. D. had delivered two of her kids in recent years. She offered a few suggestions about the layout of the patient room, but she kept going on and on about how wonderful Dr. D. was, and how much "he loved children so much".

At this point, I was ready to break and crawl through the one-way mirror. You see, Dr. D. performed several abortions per day, with a few normal deliveries thrown in during the week. Did he really love children that much?

Vaginas and Videos – Part 1

As my career in healthcare was getting started, the use of TV cameras and videotape in operating rooms was just getting underway. As time went on, videotaping surgical procedures became limited to just recording unusual cases, not routine ones.

However, when all of this "new technology" came into existence, it was like a kid getting a toy for Christmas. One such OB/GYNE doctor was the "kid". He decided that he wanted to be the first doctor in the hospital to videotape a baby being born.

He had a large medical practice and he almost always had a woman in labor. He floated the idea to several women about having their child's birth recorded. Besides the doctor...it would require a video technician to operate the equipment.

The doctor was turned down repeatedly, but eventually he talked one "mom-to-be" into allowing her baby's birth to be videotaped.

The husband was out of town and he was not going to make it back in time for the delivery, so the idea of a "video replay" sounded pretty good.

The camera and recording equipment were set up in the delivery room, everything was ready.

The vaginal birth was as normal and routine as could be. When the video was played back, the screen was filled with a close-up of the woman's vagina, and the healthy baby exiting. The new mother was excited to watch the birth of her baby. Then, a short time later, the husband returned to town and all Hell broke loose!

The purpose of the video was two-fold, one to use the video as an educational tool, and secondly, in this case, for the parents to see their child's birth. The husband went through the roof! He didn't want his wife's vagina filling the screens of TV monitors, even if the audience was only medical personnel! The doctor and video tech told him that no one would be able to identify who the mother was, and all that was seen were her "private parts."

Well, he threatened to sue the hospital and doctor for an "invasion of privacy". At that point, a signed, video consent form was produced, which included his wife's signature. At that point, he backed off and cooled down. The Hospital President got wind of this commotion, and we were ordered to erase the videotape, which we did. The husband was very happy.

The doctor in his defense later added, "Random people walking down the street couldn't see the video and exclaim, "Oh, look, that's Donna Jackson's vagina!" Stay tuned for Part 2...

Lunchtime With Kaylee

Sometimes in life, you meet people who seem to be a complete match with your personality. I worked with one such woman for 2 years. We worked on the same floor of the hospital, Kaylee, as a department secretary, and my medical media department just down the hall. Because our paths crossed frequently during the day, we would end up eating lunch together on a fairly regular basis.

Spending any time together usually resulted in both of us laughing, sometimes so much that we were crying. There wasn't any romantic chemistry or attraction between us...but we could have been a terrific comedy team. If you remember the chemistry between Regis Philbin and Kelly Ripa...then you will better understand the type of relationship we had.

Our relationship was full of fun, puns and double entendre. Many times, if we were sitting by ourselves in the employee cafeteria, we would be laughing so much that rumors started flying that we must be having an affair. Nothing could be further from the truth, but we had a lot of fun those two years we worked together.

One story involved Kaylee and her college days. She went to and graduated from Michigan State University. Her parents lived about an hour's drive away, though she lived on campus. One Friday morning she woke up and the flu bug was hitting her-hard. She felt like crap, but since the weekend was forthcoming, she decided to drive home and recuperate over the weekend.

Ah, those unexpected moments.

As she approached her home, the driveway was empty and she hit the garage door opener, parking her car inside and closing the door. She called out once she entered the home and assessed that her parents weren't there.

About that time, the flu bug was hitting her "at both ends" and she quickly made her way to the upstairs bathroom, next to her bedroom. Getting a little comfort and feeling momentarily better, she entered her room, closed the door, hopped into bed, and crawled under the covers. Just as she was feeling cozy and comfortable, she heard the front door open.

Her parents were returning home after going out for breakfast. Well, she heard her Mom and Dad coming up the stairs, using words she had never before heard from them. Apparently, her parents went out for breakfast, but came home for "dessert".

She continued to listen and soon heard the ka-ching, ka-ching noise the bed was making, as well as an expletive-filled conversation.

What was she going to do?

How could she escape the embarrassment of having heard this "interaction"?

Well, there was a family room on the lower level, and she devised a plan. She grabbed her blanket and pillow and figured out that if she laid down on the couch, covered up, and pretended to be asleep, maybe everyone could escape this embarrassment.

As she stealthily sneaked out of her room and made her way down the stairs, she had to step over clothing that hastily had been removed before her parents had made their way upstairs.

After an hour or so, the parents and their daughter ran into each other on the lower level. The parents were quite shocked to see Kaylee at home, and after hearing her explanation about coming home sick, there were some red faces, but very little conversation the whole rest of the day.

A Brief History Lesson

How many readers can identify with or have read anything significant about the year 1917? True, World War 1 was coming to an end, and the Titanic sunk in 1912, but what's the deal about 1917?

We have all heard about the Holocaust during World War 2, and many have heard about the genocide in Rwanda, but 1917 marked a period of genocide that was one of the cruelest, most vile times in world history that many have never heard of.

Turkey decided to eliminate all Armenians living in their country, as well as just killing as many Armenians as possible. There were mass shootings, hangings, children were killed, pregnant women had their babies cut out and killed-it was as horrible and gruesome as you can imagine. Sickening and disgusting-over one million Armenians perished during this "cleansing".

On more than one occasion, naked teenage girls were crucified next to each other and left to die. This period was truly an evil period that most of us have never heard of.

Fast forward to approximately 1986...

An Armenian surgeon was in an operating room looking at and reviewing x-rays of an upcoming surgery he was about to perform. The O.R. staff came shuffling in- the patient was wheeled in, next to the anesthesiologist. The surgeon looked up and all hell broke loose!

He picked up a tray of instruments and threw them at the anesthesiologist.

"Get out of here...now!"

He picked up a scalpel and threatened him. Luckily for the patient, he was under twilight sleep, and knew nothing about what was happening around him.

Now, neither the surgeon or anesthesiologist were living in 1917, but the problem was that the anesthesiologist was Turkish, the surgeon was Armenian, he was chased out of the O.R. and a new one was immediately requested. As it turns out, the surgeon had relatives killed during that "conflict"/genocide.

Operator...How Can I Help You?

As you can imagine, the telephone systems of medical centers are quite complex. When the calls come in, there is a choice of using the automated system, or staying on the line to speak to a person. The following is one such actual conversation.

"Good morning...City General, how can I help you?"

"I'm trying to get in touch with a Bernice Sexauer"

"Is she a patient?"

"No. She's a new employee".

"What department?"

"She works in the laboratories. I think she just started this week."

"You said a Bernice Sexauer, right?"

"Yes."

"Let me check. Hold on."

"Um...I can't seem to find her in the system."

"You mean you don't have any Sexauer there?"

"Sex hour? Honey we're lucky if we get a ten-minute coffee break!"

Imported Humor, or Vaginas and Videos: Part 2
Or
Not For the Squeamish Male

One of my proudest accomplishments as the head of a hospital's medical media department was to televise live surgery from our operating rooms to a major downtown hotel about 5 miles away.

It was for a national convention being held by the Association for Obstetrics and Gynecology. About 900 doctors from around the country would be attending. We had plenty of notice to figure out how to pull this off technically and logistically.

We would be using 2 operating rooms with 2 TV cameras in each room. When one case was finished, we would switch and begin televising from the 2nd room. We also needed two-way sound, so that the doctors sitting in the hotel auditorium watching the proceedings on a 30-foot screen could ask questions during surgery.

We drew block diagrams of everything we needed. It would be a terrific technical challenge, but we knew we could pull it off. One of our biggest challenges was to figure out how we would get the video and audio signals from the 3rd floor of the hospital, to the hotel 5 miles away.

Well, we decided to use microwave technology with a little help from our friends at AT&T. While we were doing this, the doctors were busy lining up and scheduling unusual surgical cases for the convention.

One of our hospital physicians had a close friend and OB Gyn doctor in Canada, and when asked if he wanted to participate at the national convention, he jumped at the chance.

Well, as the big day progressed, there were no technical difficulties and the attendees were watching unusual cases displayed on a 30-foot screen. They were asking questions back and forth, and it was all going quite smoothly.

Then, the last case of the day began. The case began with the introduction of a woman whose medical complaint was "pain upon intercourse."

Ouch.

Now usually when you hear that complaint, it means that the woman is experiencing the pain. However, in this case, it was her husband.

The Canadian physician was to tackle this final case, and he was prepared to use scopes with video cameras attached and determine what the cause of pain was.

If need be, he would use them and look at the internal female organs via laparoscopy to find out the source. Upon visual inspection, they were not finding anything unusual to cause the pain and were almost ready to give up.

The Canadian doctor persevered and refused to give up. They couldn't find out what the source of pain was, especially for her husband. They checked some prior patient notes from earlier surgeries and continued to perform a visual inspection.

The video cameras have a tiny light attached. Just then, the physician noticed a glare...a reflection of something shiny! There was a staple protruding into the vagina from a previous operation.

One of the doctors doubted that this was the source of pain.

The Canadian doctor, "Dr. Y" rebutted, "Well, how would you like it if every time you had sex with your wife, it felt like your dick was hitting a razor blade?"

Ouch!

They proceeded to remove the staple and as the saying goes...they all lived happily ever after.

The Guest Speaker Was What?

When running a hospital media department, you receive many requests for services.

One such request was to videotape a routine lecture for a particular audience. One of the female Lamaze instructors at the hospital was going to explain her services to an audience of Nursing School students.

The lecture was booked for 8 a.m. on a Monday in the hospital auditorium. It was a minor inconvenience to me, because I had to arrive early, move and set up equipment, and be ready to start at 8 a.m.

I got to work early, the equipment was set up and tested, and there I was...all alone and waiting in a rather large auditorium. Watching and waiting, I thought to myself, "Well, maybe it starts at 8:30."

At about 8:20...I tried making a few calls but got no response. I thought, "Maybe they're all on the way."

So, I waited.

About 8:45, I heard the door creak in the rear of the auditorium, and a lone nurse came in. She made her way down the stairs and asked me, "Didn't you hear?"

"About what?"

"The speaker was murdered over the weekend."

This was a shock to me, as well as to the entire hospital community. My wife and I had gone to her and used her services when we were expecting our first baby.

(The criminal was captured, and after some time, executed by lethal injection. Justice had been served, but it didn't bring back this wonderful woman and educator.)

Even Doctors Die

As we all know…good, nice people…friends and relatives…get seriously ill and die all too much. We've all seen babies and children at St. Jude's hospital, and wonder why such innocent young kids have to suffer and go through such serious trials and tribulations.

I can't imagine the emotional state of the nurses and staff when working with these kids. (And the parents!)

Besides children, even the caregivers, nurses, doctors, and auxiliary staff become ill, and sometimes die. We usually think that doctors work until an "old age", eventually retire, and we lose track of their personal lives. However, this is not always the case.

My media department and I provided services to a middle-aged cardiologist. One of his functions and responsibilities was to teach medical students, and nursing students, how to interpret heart sounds as they would listen to them through a stethoscope.

He had a machine which had a variety of pre-recorded heart sounds on it. My job was to connect or interface his machine into an auditorium sound system. The students would use headphones and plug them into headphone jacks in each of the auditorium seats.

They would listen to sounds and interpret them, as to whether they were normal or abnormal. Dr. K. taught these classes several times a year, as an introductory or refresher course.

Dr. K was one of the nicest people you could meet and work with. Unlike some, or many doctors, he would always acknowledge your presence. If you randomly passed in a hallway, he would take the time to chat with you about your job and personal life.

He was one of those people you never minded helping or providing services for. I didn't see or talk to him every day, but word spread quickly when it was learned that he was suddenly hospitalized.

Of course, being a doctor in your own hospital, and suddenly becoming a patient, gets you a lot of attention and very quickly, a lot of tests. It was a mystery at the time this all happened, but within one week, Dr. K. was no longer with us.

All we were ever told was that he contracted some virus that made his brain swell, causing him to become unconscious, and he died.

In one week, he went from being a seemingly healthy vibrant man, doctor, husband, and friend, to an "ex-member of the medical staff."

Dr. J. was a very accomplished, skilled, and a likable surgeon. He had operations scheduled several times a week, and, like most surgeons, did follow-up visits on the other days.

Having performed many gall bladder operations, he expected his patient's surgery to be fairly routine. With him in the operating room were the usual crew-scrub nurse, circulating nurse, anesthesiologist, and two surgical residents, who usually got to hold clamps during the operation, and then close-up the patient at the end by sewing or stitching.

Now whether your faith or beliefs include God, or the grim reaper, as far as life and death is concerned, there were other unforeseen plans in place for that day. At the point just when the gall bladder was removed, Dr J. paused for a moment, collapsed to the floor, and died. No known prior health issues had been recorded or documented; he simply died from cardiac arrest.

Attempts to shock him and resuscitate him were unsuccessful. Another "ex member of the medical staff."

During my career in healthcare, I've had other close associates die quickly too, like being at work on Friday, and deceased by Monday. Three of the nicest caring women I knew and worked with suffered such fate. They were all taken much too soon by breast cancer.

One woman and I exchanged children's videos all the time...and I never even knew she was sick.

One older, prominent doctor was diagnosed with an incurable, fatal disease.

Despite all the alternative painless ways to commit suicide...this doctor chose to take a swan dive from an upper floor of the hospital.

The irony of this is that they named and dedicated a conference room after him, located on the 2nd floor.

As they say, time plus tragedy equals humor.

I Didn 't Apply For This!

Julia Higgins was looking for a new job. She had a friend that worked at the hospital, who told her that there were a lot of open, non-medical positions available. The hospital had an employee turnover rate of 3% a month, which translates into a turnover rate of 36% annually-quite high.

On the right, there was a double door going directly outside. On the left, there was another door going inside the hospital to a quiet, presently un-used part of the building. There was a small elevator directly outside that door. The Human Resources department was located between these doors. There was a large sitting area with tables, so applicants could sit and fill out paper applications, if they didn't fill out one on-line.

Julia was not alone at the tables; she had obtained an application at the receptionist window and was proceeding to fill it out. Just then, a young man came in from the outside door. He was carrying a stack of medical books, rather clumsily. He was wearing a short, white coat, and wearing a stethoscope around his neck.

He set the books down for a second on Julia's table and asked her for help.

"Could you please help me take these books back to the library? It's just upstairs. It will only take a minute."

Julia thought for a moment, and then agreed. After all, she was applying for a job and wanted to seem cooperative. What happened next was a nightmare.

They split up the pile of books and walked out into the hospital hallway. He pushed the elevator button.

"The library is just up here on the second floor."

As they got off the elevator on the second floor, Julia was pushed into a room and brutally raped.

Here's the scary part.

That entire second floor right above Human Resources was totally abandoned.

There were several rooms with beds where medical residents had once used them as on-call rooms and slept at odd hours, but it hadn't been used or occupied that way for years.

My department had a storage closet on that floor, but even I only went up there a few times a year. It was deserted and kind of creepy.

Who was this person who knew that floor was abandoned, and knew that no one would hear anything, and no one would hear her cries for help?

The man ran off, Julia got herself together, went back downstairs crying, and sought help and medical attention.

She was taken right to the Emergency Room and an investigation quickly began. (The criminal was never identified and caught.)

A Sexual Interlude

At one hospital I worked at there was a physician who was a "sexologist." He was a psychiatrist, and had all the medical credentials and degrees, including a PhD.

He had a large practice, and counseled couples and individuals who had, or thought they had problems with sex. He likened himself to a local Masters and Johnson, who researched and did sex surveys in the 1950's through the 1990's.

During my time working at this hospital, my employees and I were asked to transfer dozens of movies from 16mm, to all sorts of video formats-VHS, Betamax, and later, to DVD's.

We had the equipment to do these transfers, but we could easily see what we were transferring.

Oh my!

We copied, legally by the way, sex movies that included heterosexual, gay, and even a few movies that included bestiality. Some were actually clinical and instructional, those he gave to his patients. In many cases we would just start the transfer process and turn the monitors off so we didn't have to see what was happening. Fast forward about 15 years!

I saw a story in the news about a doctor from this same institution who was arrested for having inappropriate sexual relations with his patients. Who do you immediately think came to mind?

Much to my surprise and my fellow employees' surprise, it wasn't him!

Turns out it was a dentist, who would suggest more than a shot for anesthesia, and while his female patients were unconscious...well let's just say that this dentist proceeded to fill the wrong cavity!

Food For Thought

As you can imagine, hospitals prepare thousands of meals per day for patients, employees, and visitors. The Food Service department is busy 24/7 and is one of the largest departments in a hospital.

In fact, hospitals have competitions, where meals are submitted to judges who rank them. This has served to improve the quality of patient food over the years. I once worked at a small hospital who beat out larger teaching hospitals for first place-kind of like David vs. Goliath.

Food Service departments usually have 2 or 3 shifts of employees, which is an inconvenience to people, but they are usually paid a shift differential for their time and effort.

Juan Rodriquez had been a faithful, reliable employee over the years and had worked his way up to Supervisor of the day shift, which was the busiest of the day. He placed orders for food, did employee scheduling, and had to work on menu selection on a weekly basis, as well as day to day.

In the department work area, the Shift Supervisor had a large glass office in the middle of the department. This enabled them sight lines to all the different areas of the department.

In recent weeks, there had been some employee turnover, and to cover vacancies, schedules had to be adjusted. Some were asked to move to a different shift, or in some cases, work 2 shifts if they wanted to. Juan had called a staff meeting and told his employees of this necessary, but temporary situation. He wasn't aware of any grumbling or complaining.

Juan started his shift about 5:30 a.m. and worked until mid-afternoon. After about three weeks into this new period, and new time schedule, Juan made his way from the parking lot to his office. He was mentally planning and laying out his agenda for the day in his mind.

As he entered his office and approached his desk, he noticed something a little "out of place", like a butcher knife firmly planted into the seat of his chair!

He called security right away-they took a picture and questioned employees working in that area.

They were surprised as well, and nobody had seen anyone going into or leaving the office.

Was this a joke or prank of some kind?

About 8:30, when the Administrator got to work, he was made aware of the situation.

He called meetings of all three shifts. All employees were told that if they had any problems or grievances, to call him directly and they would be discussed. Not one meeting was scheduled.

Two weeks went by, and when Juan approached his office...he was very cautious. After all, you don't come to work every day expecting to find a large knife protruding from your chair. He dismissed the incident as a prank and was starting to relax and put the incident behind him.

Monday morning, at 5:45 a.m. Juan drove to work, entered his office and was putting some work he had taken home on his desk.

All of a sudden, he heard the door close behind him and lock. There, between Juan and the door, stood one of his employees holding a large butcher knife.

In the middle of this glass office, with employees working nearby, the assailant immediately attacked Juan. The noise and screams immediately got the other employees' attention and they horrifically knew what was happening.

Someone called the operator and security right away. Others threw chairs and objects at the glass windows trying to distract the intruder or break the glass so they could try and assist Juan.

Armed security guards arrived on the scene with guns drawn. The assailant was sitting on Juan's desk, and Juan's bloody body was on the floor.

Security unlocked the door and immediately took the dazed assailant into custody.

A few moments later the local police arrived. In the meantime, an emergency room crew arrived on the scene and tended to Juan. It was too late.

During the struggle Juan's carotid artery was severed and there was a fatal wound to his chest. There were attempts to help by the ER team, but it was too late.

As it turns out, the perpetrator was indeed a food service employee...an employee with an addiction to cocaine, and a bad attitude about the shift/schedule changes. It was an easy quick trial; there were plenty of witnesses and he was found guilty and sentenced to life imprisonment.

As a follow—up, they looked at the assailant's employee record. He had gotten good annual reviews at the hospital for about three years. The Administrator who oversaw the Food Service department was subsequently fired. Whew!

Ahhhhh...Live TV

Long before Face Time, Skype and streaming videos, many large companies would disseminate information via teleconferences. These were companies who had branches around the country and needed to have immediate interaction between themselves. The major auto companies did this, as well as large medical associations.

One company I worked for was televising such an event. There was a female host/moderator and a few panelists. The presentation went from the parent company's TV studio up to a satellite, and then down from the satellite to all of the branches. At the conclusion of the "lecture", employees from the branches could call a central number and ask questions.

The female moderator would take the call, and the panelists would respond. After a few routine calls, a new call came in: "Hi, I would just like to say that we have quite an attractive moderator today, and she fills out her sweater quite nicely." A panelist jumped in and said, "We appreciate your call and compliments, and now let's get onto the next question."

After that, the calls were answered off-camera and the questions were written out and handed to the moderator.

It's All-Star Baseball Time!

Large hospitals have many different places for employees to change their clothes and slip into uniforms. During shift changes they can become quite crowded for a short time.

These locker rooms are not typically located in patient care areas. (Thankfully, in this case.)

During all this interaction...interesting things occur, such as drugs exchanging hands, and gambling on sporting events.

I have personally seen large amounts of money changing hands.

One guy pulled out a rubber-banded roll of bills that was quite impressive!

It was the day before the baseball All-Star game in July and there was all sorts of betting going on.

Bets were made on how many innings a pitcher would last, the final score, and how many home runs would be hit.

Bets were placed on almost anything.

Well, the day after the All-Star game, an employee lost a bet and didn't have the money on him to pay up.

His "debt collector" said nothing, reached into his pocket, pulled out a 22-caliber handgun and shot him in the leg!

He then calmly disappeared out of the locker room and hospital. Other employees helped the shooting victim up to the Emergency Room, where he was promptly taken care of.

Luckily, no arteries were hit, and the wound was non-life threatening.

The shooter was arrested at his home and never worked at the hospital again.

That Will Be 100 Dollars

The kind of department I managed had a large variety of audio-visual and video equipment. Before video took over, there were 16mm movies distributed for education and training. The movies were loaded onto Bell & Howell 16mm projectors and presented at meetings. My department had several of these.

One morning, a young man came into my office carrying a Bell & Howell box. He said it had a new projector in it and wanted to know if I wanted to buy it for $100. He worked in the Transportation department, which moves patients around the hospital for tests and such, and then takes them back to their rooms. The price immediately caught my attention, because it was very cheap, and the projector was indeed brand new. I couldn't help but think that perhaps this was stolen.

The security office was located around the corner from my area, and I had a good working relationship with one of the investigators. I approached him, he took the model number and serial number, and said he would get back to me. Indeed, it was stolen, it was reported missing from a railroad boxcar that had been broken into.

Security called the employee down and he was suspended for a few days. As it turned out, this young man and his friends had many of these in their possession. There was ultimately a court date set, and the railroad police were going to produce the evidence, and I would have to testify.

This made me nervous because the employee had not been fired, and the idea of running into him at work was a little scary. I was concerned about retaliation.

Well, the court date came, the railroad police picked me up, and off to court we went. I was nervous because I was going to have to testify that a fellow employee tried to sell me "hot" merchandise.

Thank God for plea deals.

The case was called, the two lawyers approached the bench, and the employee/defendant was fined $100, that's it, case over.

No testifying for me.

It was interesting that the hospital did not fire the employee. I saw him just once after that and he was thankful that the case was settled as a misdemeanor and only a fine.

I was glad there was no hostility or retaliation, after all, it was my doing that he was arrested.

I Just Wanna Go On My Cruise
Or
Theft, Race and Lie–Detectors

My department had a large inventory of equipment-audio-visual equipment, video cameras and recorders...a plethora of hardware.

It was a Friday night.

My wife and I lived about 23 miles from the medical complex where I worked. We were looking forward to a winter cruise coming up in two weeks. The idea of a Caribbean cruise in the middle of winter seemed like a wonderful idea.

Since it was Friday and a payday, we decided to splurge and go out for dinner. While we were enjoying a nice meal, 23 miles away a theft was taking place. One of my employees was seen loading some of my departments' equipment into a van.

When I returned to work on Monday, I noticed right away that there were some items missing, and my employee had called in sick. There had been a note left for me, in which an employee stated he saw a van being loaded with equipment.

I reported the situation to the Security office, and

it was turned over to one of their investigators. Well, they decided to question my employee and myself. I told them that during the time that the theft was taking place, I was out to dinner with my wife. I even still had the restaurant receipt!

The security manager thought we should BOTH take a lie detector/polygraph test. Being the department manager, I strongly protested. After all, Employee X was seen loading equipment into a van!

"Well, because your employee is of a different race and culture, we can't have it look like we are racially discriminating."

They called in an outside company who routinely performs polygraph tests, and they scheduled it for two weeks later - the time I was supposed to be on my cruise. Not only did I have nothing to do with the theft, they were interfering with my scheduled vacation time!

Well, they rescheduled my test, and I passed. Employee X, not so much. He was suspended, and I left on my long-awaited cruise. While I was gone, the missing equipment mysteriously re-appeared, and Employee X had been fully re-instated! As an aftermath, Employee X was fired by me at a later date. He was found buying equipment and charging it to the hospital.

Computers and Medicine

One of my responsibilities was to maintain and keep the computer lab up and functioning 24/7. It was located in the medical library, which was adjacent to my office.

There were a large variety of medical CDs, DVDs, as well as complete access to the internet.

The computers were accessible to medical and nursing students, medical residents, and attending physicians. After hours, the computer lab was accessible via a key card.

Upon my arrival one morning, I saw something on the PC monitors that had never been there before-pornography. I cleared and restarted the computers-problem solved. I put a sign up that said that the computers were to be used for medical research only. I also told my boss, who was the Director of Medical Education. He suggested that we install on-line filters so that the porno websites would be inaccessible. Well, you can block websites, but not block body part names-after all, this is a medical and healthcare field. There are always ways to get around the filters.

Well, we set up a hidden security camera, built into a clock. The offender was quickly caught.

He was a married resident with children, who lived across the street. He would come over at night, while on call, and entertain himself when not looking after patients. He was reprimanded and reminded that if really necessary, he could entertain himself at home.

Bucking Bronco?

Let's face it...you don't hear the word "Bucking" very much anymore. I always thought it was connected to rodeos, not medicine.

My very first surgery to videotape, I was a little concerned. I didn't know if I would get queasy and pass out or what to expect.

A young, twenty-something woman was to have surgery on her cheek. Turns out she had a tumor of the salivary gland. I set up the camera/recorder and was ready to go. The doctor took a marker out and drew a line on her cheek. She was unconscious and the surgeon was ready to start.

As he started his incision, it was like a scene from the Exorcist. Her body started shaking and seemed to be rising off the operating room table. The doctor stopped for a moment. Though she was semi-unconscious, the anesthesiologist had not given her enough anesthesia. Her body was responding to the cutting and pain.

He quickly administered more and everything settled down. I quickly learned this "phenomena" is called "bucking" in the medical realm. She had no memory of the incident, the tumor was benign and removed, and she was fine.

Election Night Terror

It was a typical November Presidential Election night. The TV viewing that night consisted of nothing but election night news, results and constant updates.

While the country was electing a new leader, 3 nurses working in the ICU couldn't wait until their shift was over. One patient had died, and the others required constant monitoring, medicine updates and changes. Eleven o'clock couldn't come soon enough.

Sandy was a personal neighbor of mine. She was in her twenties, single, and a super-nice, caring person. She was well-suited for being a nurse. She was an attractive blond, who usually wore her hair in a ponytail, which was a good style for working in the Intensive Care Unit.

The trio of nurses decided that at the end of their shift, they would go out for a quick drink or two, split a pizza and unwind. Sandy and her co-workers clocked out and proceeded to a local establishment about a mile away. All three nurses rode together that night because one of the three was lucky enough to find a parking spot just outside the hospital on the street.

After sharing a pizza and a couple of beverages, they split the bill and drove back to the hospital. The driver pulled up to the Security Office, dropped Sandy and the other nurse off, and drove away. The hospital security department had a personal safety policy in place, but Sandy and her co-worker were not going to benefit from it tonight.

At the change of shift, especially and most importantly at night, an employee could request that a security officer would accompany them to their cars in the parking garage. The "officer" told Sandy and Carol that normally he would be happy to walk with them to their cars, but he refused because the policy said that it was no longer the "change-of shift" time frame, but two hours past. The two weren't very happy about that, so they protested and decided to complain the next day.

They proceeded to walk the two blocks to the garage. It was dark, windy, chilly and quiet, with the temperature hovering just about 30 degrees. The only noise was their uniform shoes hitting the pavement with each step. It was quiet...almost too quiet.

In retrospect, when they reached the garage, they should have stayed together, retrieved one car, and then dropped the other at her car, but for whatever reason, they didn't. Carol was on a lower level of the garage. The two said goodnight and she exited.

Sandy had three more floors to go and hurriedly pushed the button for her floor again.

A cold shiver hit her, and she was anxious to get out of the cold. The elevator door opened and she moved briskly towards her car. A gust of wind blew through the garage, and she was coldly reminded that winter was just around the corner. Unfortunately, something evil was lurking just around the corner too.

Sandy removed her car keys from her coat pocket and proceeded to unlock her door.

"Hi."

Before she could open the door, she was pushed hard against the car, and she knew this couldn't be good. Her assailant turned her around, reached inside and hit the door-lock button, unlocking all four doors.

She tried kneeing him in the groin, but she missed. This only pissed off her assailant. He reached behind his back and brandished a knife. He pushed her towards the back door of the car and shoved her inside face-down. Sandy screamed and he retaliated by swinging the knife and slicing her ear.

She felt the warmth of her blood and wondered how bad her injury was. She knew what was happening, and she felt her clothes being tugged at, and semi-removed. Then the unthinkable happened. She cried and screamed simultaneously...but to no avail.

There was just no one around to hear her cries for help. While she laid on the back seat, face-down, bleeding and crying, the assailant exited the car and grabbed the keys from the front seat.

"Get out! Now!"

She tried to pull herself together, as her hair was being pulled, and she was being pushed towards the rear of the car. The man was fidgeting with the keys, but he couldn't open the trunk.

"Open this!"

Sandy got the trunk open and her life quickly flashed before her eyes. She knew if she got in, she was going to be taken somewhere and killed.

"Get in!"

Sandy mustered all her courage, thoughts, and energy simultaneously, and threw the car keys as far away as she could.

"Bitch, get in!"

He forcibly pushed her in the trunk and closed the lid.

"I'll be right back!"

Sandy was hoping she threw the keys far enough

away that he wouldn't find them. She was still trying to catch her breath, while simultaneously waiting for this monster to return. She knew that at any moment she could be driven out of the garage and killed somewhere.

Darkness, cold and solitude were setting in. Several minutes had gone by. She waited for the monster. She felt her ear. It hurt…but the bleeding must have stopped. She heard nothing outside. It was 3 a.m. and no one was coming or going into or out of the parking garage. It was cold, and half of her clothes were gone. It was total darkness in the trunk.

She felt around and found the backside of the back seat. She pushed with her hands, but nothing budged. She tried to position herself to push with her legs and feet, but still nothing moved.

Sandy felt herself getting weak. She also was becoming very tired. On top of everything, she was still concerned that her attacker may re-appear. She told herself that if she fell asleep, she would freeze and die. Groping around the trunk in total darkness, she found something - a blanket! A blanket was still in the trunk from trips to the beach!

She wrapped herself in the beach blanket as best as she could. "They will find me like a dead, frozen burrito!", she mused.

As she wiggled around to try and get warm and somewhat comfortable, she felt something cold. She reached for it and determined it must be the lug-nut wrench.

Sandy paused for a minute. She wanted to start pounding on the trunk of the car, but what if her assailant heard it and returned? She listened. Silence. No cars coming or going. Total blackness and total silence. She pounded a few times-nothing. She paused to collect her thoughts. Damn, my ear is hurting, she thought to herself.

She told herself if she could make it, the change of shift should be coming up. She would only start pounding when she heard something. She thought for a moment, "Is there enough air in here? Am I gonna suffocate?"

She realized and convinced herself that car trunks are not air-tight and that would be one less way for her to die. She felt herself shiver and then she heard something! It sounded like a car. She began pounding - nothing. She collected her thoughts. "It's cold out. Incoming cars would have their windows rolled up, heaters and radios going. No one will hear me."

Just then...she had an epiphany.

Another car passed by. "I'll wait 'til I hear someone walking or talking, then I'll start pounding".

She was so tired, but the excitement of that idea gave her renewed courage and energy. Time passed. Another car. She listened. Nothing. "Change of shift must be coming soon!", she hoped.

Out of nowhere, she heard voices. She began pounding and screaming, "Help, help!"

"What the hell's going on?"

"Please get me out of here!"

"Alright, I'm gonna run and get help. I'll be right back."

It seemed like an eternity. She heard voices again, getting closer.

"She's in here!"

Sandy heard loud noises...drilling, pounding, and then suddenly the brightness of sunlight! Sandy was helped out of the trunk. They placed her into a wheelchair. She saw two maintenance guys, a nurse and an ER doctor. She heard a siren and then a city police car pulled into the parking garage.

In the aftermath of this horrific incident, Sandy was wheeled into the ER, warmed up, and then the staff followed the protocol for treating a rape victim. She was asked a plethora of questions, and no, she couldn't give a definitive description of her attacker.

Epilogue...

Sandy explained the whole story several times. The security officer that wouldn't escort the nurses to their car was fired. A lawsuit was filed and Sandy received a modest settlement. She resigned her position as a nurse, kept in touch with her friends, and re-located to a smaller suburban hospital, to start a new life.

(Note: Cell phones did not exist at the time of this incident, nor did all cars have inside trunk release levers.)

Dr. Death

My wife enjoyed working in the Special Care Nursery, most of the time. The nursery is comprised of many pre-mature babies fighting for their lives, hoping to make it into a normal existence.

Let's just say that if you are ever hospitalized and hear your doctor state that he/she is going to get "Aggressive" with your treatment...RUN FOR YOUR LIFE!

My wife took care of this tiny, little baby who did have some medical issues, one of which was difficulty breathing. He slept most of the time, but if you spent time and talked to him, he would open his eyes and give you a smile that would touch your heart.

Whenever I had time, I visited my wife and this baby, who we shall call MLB. My wife was right, his smile was infectious.

One morning, upon starting her shift, during "report", this female doctor said she was going to get "aggressive" with MLB's treatment. What this ultimately resulted in was MLB's death. My wife heard her state she was going to administer a drug that would slow down MLB's respiratory rate.

"You're going to give this to a baby who already has compromised breathing?", my wife protested.

The doctor rattled off her justification for this and said was going to do it the next morning.

Well, my wife was on the verge of calling the police...but she didn't.

You don't have to be an expert to know what was about to happen.

The next day the doctor gave this drug to the baby, and lo and behold, MLB suffered respiratory arrest and died. If you are having difficulty breathing and you are given a drug to inhibit respiration...what the hell did they think was going to happen?

To this day, my wife feels that "Dr. Death" murdered this little defenseless baby. She cried many times discussing this case. I can still see the smile of that helpless baby.

Triplets? Maybe Not!

My wife experienced this as a nurse.

There was one patient who thoroughly disgusted the entire nursing staff.

An expectant patient came in, and after an ultrasound was done, you could clearly see that there were three distinct "fetuses" in her uterus. She was having triplets!

She was admitted as a patient, but there was a lot of subdued info about this patient. Her doctor wasn't sharing much information. Then it leaked out.

The mother decided she could only handle and support two children...not three. The doctor basically said, "No problem, we'll just take one away."

Using ultrasound, he systematically inserted a long needle through the women's abdomen and into the uterus. The needle was guided into the baby's heart, potassium was injected, and that baby's heart stopped beating. Now there were two.

The "mother" was released. Everyone was disgusted with the mother AND her doctor. About two weeks went by, and the nurses saw that this woman was being re-admitted.

She just decided that she didn't want to be pregnant anymore.

So, she went from having triplets to not being pregnant at all.

Wouldn't birth control have been much easier?

I Don't Feel So Good

As previously mentioned, my "Educational Television Services" department provided a wide variety of video services to the teaching hospital.

We received a call from a physician who wanted us to record him demonstrating new surgical instruments. My female co-worker, Carol, scheduled a date and time, and we were all set.

We were going to use two video cameras, one set up on the side for a "wide-shot/overview", and I would be at the foot of the operating room table and provide close-up shots of the instruments. We videotaped everywhere in the hospital and our location today would be out-patient surgery.

We had the cameras all set up and we were waiting to record. A nurse walked the female patient into the room and got her situated on the operating room table. Dr. M. then walked in with a small tray of instruments, covered by a towel. As he uncovered them, he wanted to make sure I could clearly show them and get close-up shots.

He gave the patient an injection into her vagina, and, at about the same time, the nurse asked the young woman if she would like her to hold her hand, which is unusual for us to hear.

the patient said "yes", and at about the same exact time, Carol and my eyes met, and we instantaneously knew what was about to happen. There were six living entities in that room, and only five were to exit alive!

The realization hit us, and Carol turned white as a ghost. She excused herself from the operating room. I hated this too, but it was an early-stage abortion with what they call a vacuum curettage.

The doctor inserted these new instruments through the cervix into the uterus, moved them vigorously around, then connected the suction machine. A combination of blood and fluids came out, and it was all over.

Another dead baby. (Excuse me, fetus). All in a day's work.

(My co-worker, Carol, was found sitting outside the room with her head down between her knees, recovering from almost passing out.)

One Number Off Can Make or Break Your Entire Day

Empathy.

If you know what this is...you probably have it. It's the ability to identify with or experience the thoughts, feeling or attitudes of others. So, as you read this next story, try to ask yourself how you would feel and react.

If you were one number off on a winning lottery ticket, you'd be disappointed. Here's another example of how being one number off, could just ruin your day.

John and I worked at the same hospital for a number of years. We were in different departments, but our paths crossed quite frequently. We became close friends. We would go out to our favorite buffet restaurant together and he was even a groomsman in my wedding.

At one point, he decided to accept a job at another hospital about 2 miles away. Within the first week of his new employment, he was called into his new supervisor's office. He was told he was being suspended until an investigation was thoroughly completed about his credentials. John was understandably shocked and bewildered.

All that he was told was that there was a problem with the background check that was done.

When you apply for jobs at hospitals and schools, the company routinely completes a background check on you. They won't hire you if you have a criminal record. It's just too much of a risk.

One of the easier ways for the employer to do this is through the State Police. When you apply, your employer usually asks you for your driver's license number, and they check with the records of the State Police.

Well, my friend John had quite a background! I didn't know that he had spent several years at a downstate prison facility for selling and distributing major amounts of illegal drugs!

How would you feel and react if this is what YOU were confronted with?

His new employer told him they had his prison record. John protested and told them that this is a mistake, and to just call his former hospital, (and me). For whatever reason, they simply refused to do this. They told him that they would run another background check, and they bitched about the fact that this would cost another $200.

Well, the second background check came back just fine. He was allowed to come back to work and received back pay for the time he was suspended.

So, what had happened?

The State Police clerk typed the wrong number into her computer and this resulted in the misinformation and suspension.

And it was all because of typing one wrong number by mistake!

Call John Wayne!

In an area of the city, where I once worked, there was a large Native-American segment of the population. On a weekend night, in the Emergency Room, most of the attending physicians were off and it was staffed by residents and medical students.

An ambulance rolled in, and the patient was a large male Native-American, who was obviously intoxicated. As if that were not bad enough, there was an arrow sticking out of him!

Luckily for him, it was stuck in his waist, from front to back, near the fatty part of his side. The arrow had not hit any organs and was not life-threatening. the resident wasn't sure how to handle this removal. He called an attending physician and asked how he should handle this. The direct quote and first advice was: "Put the wagons in a circle!"

A Hymen and an Oil Change

One of my many "jobs" was to take pictures or videos of unusual patient cases.

Julie was a pleasant, 14 year-old-girl, going through puberty, with all the changes that a typical teen-ager would go through.

She was beginning to experience menstruation and there was an issue that needed to be resolved. Her hymen had never been broken, and rather than being a fairly weak tissue covering the inside entrance to the vagina, her hymen was more like the Great Wall of China. Her vagina was completely closed and nothing was going in or out!

With menstruation ensuing...this was a problem that needed to be resolved. Her doctor decided to use a laser to make a vertical incision into the hymen. Julie was under general anesthesia and the doctor moved the laser into position.

If you have ever seen your car get an oil change, you can picture what happens when you take the plug out of the oil pan. A strong, steady stream of oil pours out of the pan.

Well, when the laser penetrated the hymen, let's just say, "It was a gusher!"

A steady stream of blood, clots, and fluid poured out! It took several minutes for the draining to stop. After that, she was thoroughly cleaned out, and hopefully everything returned to normal.

During the procedure, the laser tech commented, "Whatever happened to the old-fashioned way of breaking a hymen?" In Julie's case, that method wouldn't have worked.

An Alley and a Carpet

One of the hospitals I worked at was a terrific neighborhood hospital. Great co-workers, dedicated staff, wonderful place to work. However, the area is one of the poorest in the city. People live on the streets and some suffer from mental illness.

On a cold winter night, a homeless man needed to keep warm. In an alley not too far from the hospital, he saw that someone had thrown away quite a bit of carpeting. He rolled the carpeting up and slid down inside it. But there was a problem that would cost him his life.

Sometime while the man was sleeping, he moved from being along the edge of the alley, towards the middle. Totally unaware of this...he was run over by a garbage truck.

The men on the truck realized that they had rolled over something unusual, and when they saw what happened they immediately called the police and an ambulance. There was nothing that could be done to save him. He was literally squished to death in his sleep.

A Weenie Roast

Glen Parsons met a group of his friends once a month, on a Tuesday night. Glen and his four friends went to school together and stayed in touch over the years. They all had a variety of different jobs, but they would meet once a month, share pizza and pitchers of beer, catch up, and then proceed home to their families.

Glen didn't live too far away, so he would just hop on the train for a short ride home. One night as he went upstairs to the train platform, a familiar urge hit him. He remembered he should have used the restroom before he left the pizza joint. He looked everywhere for a restroom, even though he knew that there weren't any.

Well, nature was calling, and since there wasn't anyone else on the platform...he decided to answer the call...with a split-second decision that would forever change his life. Unable to hold it any longer, he proceeded to pee off the platform, which turned out to be an electrifying mistake. His urine made a steady stream, where it met the infamous electrified "third rail", which carries the power for the train. In a flash, Glen was electrocuted, burned badly, and died. Certainly, a tragedy.

Luckily for me, I was not asked to "Grab your camera and come to the E.R."

Generosity Gone Bad

One hospital had a clinic for people who were uninsured with little income.

The clinic was small and only open certain hours throughout the week. There were no charges for services.

Certain doctors would volunteer their time and it was a nice way to help the community.

A long-standing resident and member of the community would donate a rather large amount of money on an annual basis. When he would make his donation, he would present one of those large checks to the hospital president.

I was always called to take a picture of the check presentation. In the meantime, this local donor had moved out of state, but he would always come back to make his donation.

Well, the unscrupulous hospital president accepted the six-figure check, and soon after the donor had left town, he permanently closed the clinic, and the money vanished along with the clinic.

Bodies, Autopsies and Cadavers...Oh, My!

Whether you are a nursing student or medical student, or even a student in some advanced high school biology classes, you will have the experience of working with the bodies of deceased human beings.

Usually, there is a preliminary class beforehand, and the instructor will have a few things to share before you actually begin your "lab" work.

You will be told, and rightfully so...these bodies were once living people, who were babies and loved by their parents, and you should have respect for the people whose bodies you will be handling.

On the other hand, as to not scare you, you will also be told about natural gases present in the bodies, and by moving the body around, there may be some =strange, but funny sounds emitted from almost any orifice on the body, and although it can be scary...it is ok to laugh.

Where There's Smoke...There's Asthma!

When you are part of a hospital department, or manage a non-medical department, you are often asked to be part of a committee.

One gentleman was retiring, and I was asked by the hospital administration if I wanted to become the "Head of the Fire Safety Committee." After reviewing the duties, I decided that it sounded like a fun opportunity.

I had to conduct a minimum of three fire drills per quarter, on each shift, with a total of 12 per year. I had a red "Mars" light and I could choose any area of the hospital to conduct a drill.

I never gave anyone a heads up on where the drill would take place. I would walk into an area, turn the light on, and announce there was a fire. I was aided by assistants to watch, time and document whether the correct procedure was followed by the staff. I didn't mind doing this at all, but it did involve coming in early or staying late and conducting the drills.

In addition, I was responsible for other activities throughout the year. For example, during Fire Prevention Week in October, the committee and I would sell Black & Decker smoke detectors during lunchtime. I was amazed at how many we sold to the employees.

Nancy, a nurse who assisted me, came up with an idea for a different kind of fire drill. This new kind of drill would take place in the basement of the hospital where there were several departments. There were no patients in the basement, but there was the Pharmacy, Medical Records, Housekeeping, Telecommunications and a few other departments.

Nancy wanted to host a fire drill scenario with a little more realism. We rented a fog machine, and the idea was to fill the basement with fog/smoke, and then announce the drill. We decided our "target" area would be Medical Records.

To create the fog, you pour a special liquid into the fog machine. The liquid heats up, a fan turns on, and the fog is distributed where ever you want it to go. In addition to the flashing Mars light, I decided I would turn on a theatrical light I had, with a red gel covering the lens of the light. The light gave the smoke a red glow and I must admit it looked pretty cool.

Nancy and I proceeded to fill the wing of the basement with fog. I then opened the door to Medical Records, set the red, flashing Mars light down, and announced there was a problem/fire. Well, there was never a fire drill held down there before, and the employees started scrambling around looking for the sheets with the correct protocol to follow.

Some staff members saw the red fog and became a little "panicky", so we reminded them this was just a drill and there was no actual threat or real fire.

There was a lot of documentation going on for this one!

We turned the fog machine off, turned on some large, portable fans to disperse the fog, and it was all over...well...almost.

Nancy and I were clueless that fog machines and their chemical output can cause an asthma-like reaction in certain people.

Several employees, including myself, found ourselves with a lingering cough for several minutes.

The fog created a "tickle" reaction in our throats, resulting in the cough response.

Nancy and I looked at the label on the bottle of "liquid fog" and there was a tiny disclaimer which we didn't see (Really!) that said: "May cause some people to have a cough-like reaction".

Well, that was the last time she and I decided to get quite that creative!

Thankfully...nobody was harmed during our fire drill experiment! All in a day's work at *City General!*

Meet Tom Orcutt

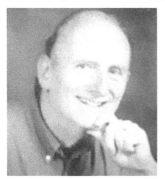

Tom Orcutt is a first-hand expert regarding the secrets held between hospital floors and walls.

The author and his wife worked a combined 40 years in the healthcare industry.

Orcutt wrote and produced hundreds of medical publications and educational videos for the healthcare industry, many of which have won awards.

The author will continue to create new publications for your enjoyment and enlightenment.

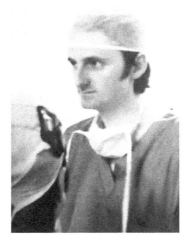

Made in USA - Kendallville, IN
1187077_9781735048505
10.28.2020 0905